Delicious Sugar Free Recipes that Have Nothing to Do With Sugar!

An Impressive No Sugar Cookbook!

Table of Contents

Introduction

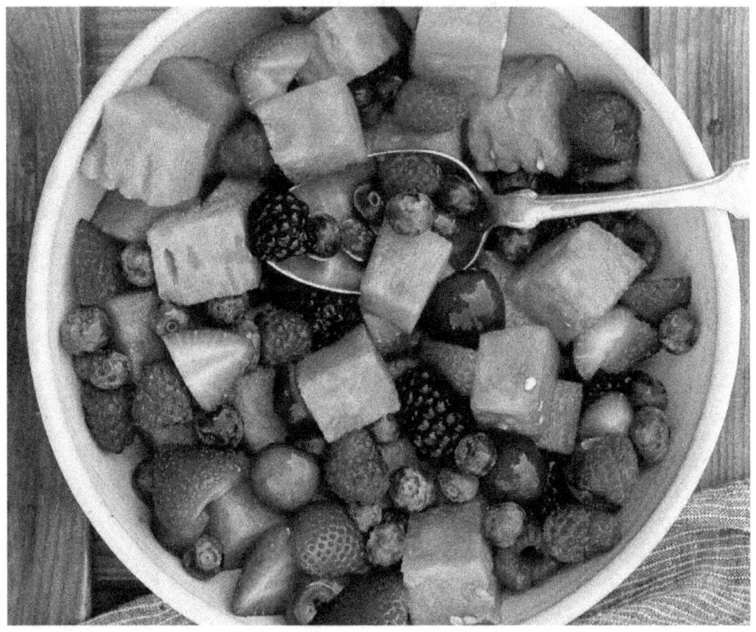

One of the questions that I get most times is "what else is there to enjoy if I don't eat or drink sugary things?". And I always get to reply, "everything else that is not sugary!!"

Then the next question is "what else is their asides from sugary meals?", and that is where I whip out this recipe book!

This recipe book is nothing like you have seen before!! This recipe book features meals that would not make you miss sugary meals at all!

This recipe book is here to make your non-sugary lifestyle worth it!!

So, flip the pages and let's start with our delicious pancake recipe!!!

1. Grilled Beef with Pineapple Marinade

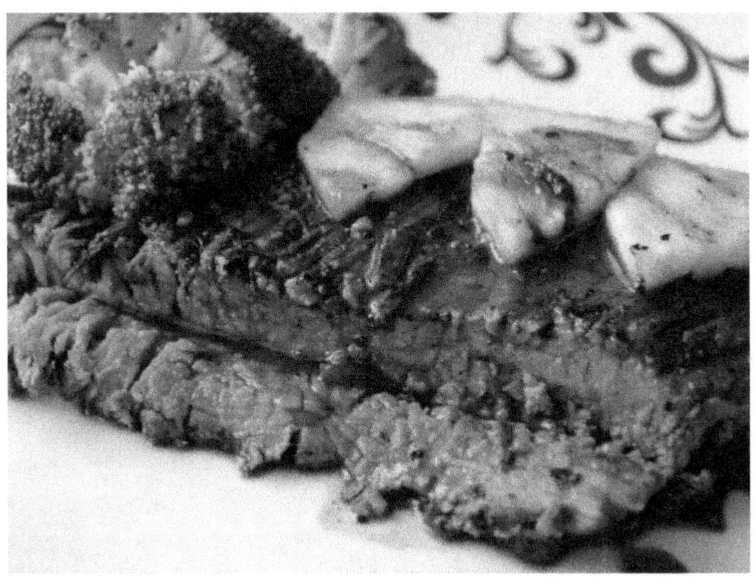

Preparation time: 25 minutes

Yield: 4 servings

The list of ingredients:

- 1 teaspoon ginger paste
- 1 teaspoon sea salt
- 2 oz. beef steaks
- 1 teaspoon garlic paste
- 1/2 cup pineapple

- 2 tablespoons lemon juice

- 2 tablespoons coconut oil

- 1 cup pineapple juice

Methods:

A. In a blender, add the pineapple, oil, lemon juice, pineapple juice, salt, ginger paste, and garlic paste then blend well.
B. Pour this mixture on the steaks and rub it in using your hands.
C. Cover and place in the fridge for 10-15 minutes.
D. Preheat the grill and grease it with oil.
E. Place the steaks on the heated grill and cook until nicely browned on both sides.
F. Serve and enjoy.

2. Green, Curried Spinach

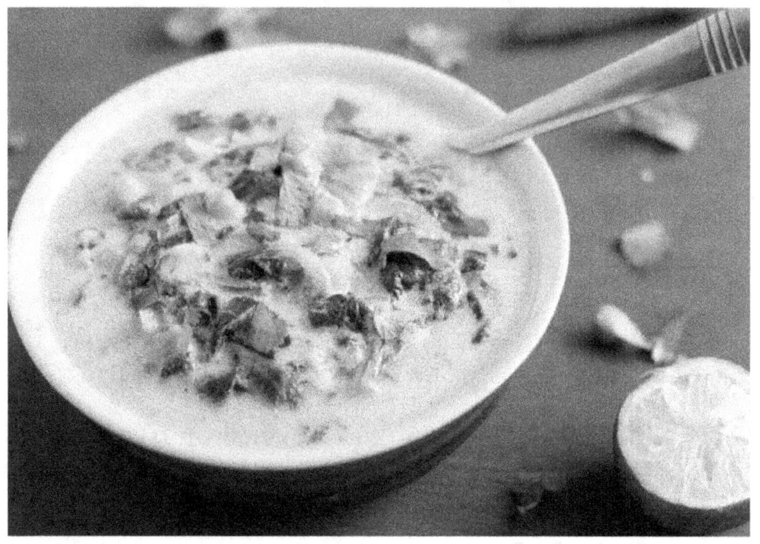

Preparation time: 30 minutes

Yield: 5 servings

The list of ingredients:

- 2 cups chicken broth
- 2-inch ginger root (shredded)
- 1 tablespoon coconut oil
- 1 teaspoon garlic paste
- 1 green chili
- 1/4 teaspoon turmeric powder

- 1/2 cup water

- 1/4 teaspoon salt

- 2 cups spinach leaves (chopped)

Methods:

A. In a blender, add the spinach, water, and green chili then blend until smooth.

B. Heat the oil in a pan and add the ginger and garlic, sautéing for 1 minute.

C. Add the spinach and fry for 5 minutes or until its color changes slightly.

D. Pour in the chicken broth and add the salt. Cook on a low heat for 15-20 minutes.

E. Serve and enjoy.

3. Lamb Stew

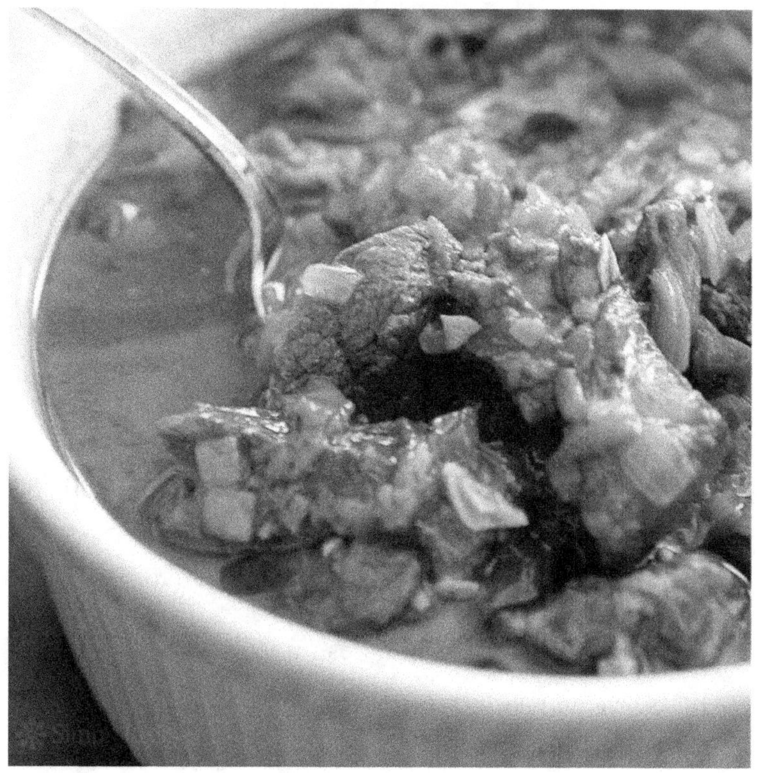

Preparation time: 10 minutes

Yield: 3 servings

The list of ingredients:

- 3-4 garlic cloves
- 1 teaspoon chili powder
- 2 tablespoons vinegar

- 1/2 teaspoon salt
- 2 tablespoons olive oil
- 1/2 teaspoon cinnamon powder
- 1 oz. lamb meat (boiled)
- 1 onion (sliced)
- 1/2 teaspoon cumin powder
- 1 cup tomato puree
- 1/4 teaspoon turmeric powder
- 1 cup vegetable broth

Methods:

A. Heat the oil in a pan, add the onion, and cook until lightly golden.
B. Add the boiled lamb and fry for 10 minutes.
C. Add the tomato puree, salt, chili powder, turmeric powder, and vinegar and fry for 5 minutes on high heat.
D. Add the vegetable broth and leave to cook on low heat for 15 minutes.
E. Add the cumin powder and cinnamon powder then remove from the heat.
F. Serve and enjoy.

4. Watermelon, Mint, and Feta Salad

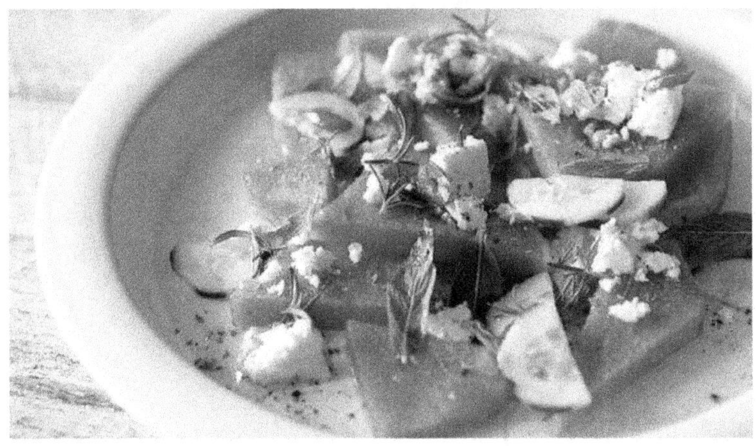

Preparation time: 15

Yield: 2 servings

The list of ingredients:

- 1/2 cup orange juice
- 2 tablespoons lemon juice
- 1 tablespoon freshly chopped mint leaves
- 1 watermelon (diced)
- 2 tablespoons brown sugar
- 1/4 cup feta cheese (crumbled)

Methods:

A. In a bowl, add the orange juice, brown sugar, lemon juice, and mint leaves then mix well.

B. In a serving bowl, add the watermelon and the orange juice mixture.

C. Serve and enjoy.

5. Citrus Pick-Me-Up

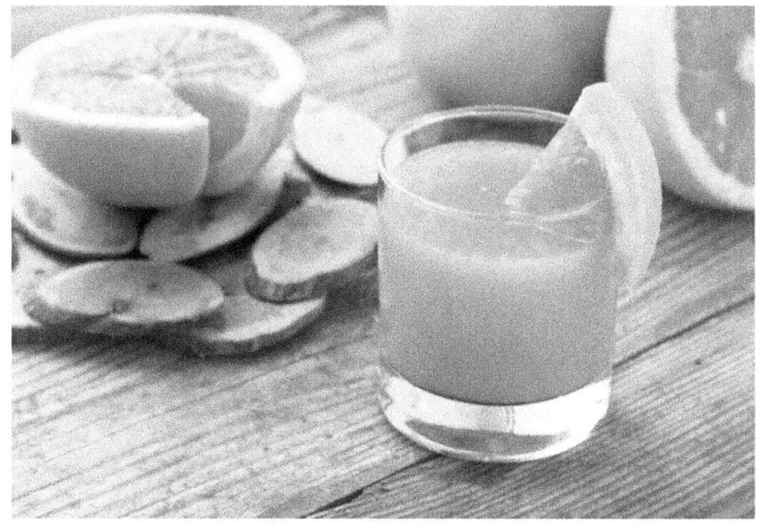

Preparation time: 5

Yield: 2 servings

The list of ingredients:

- 3 oranges (peeled)
- 1 tablespoon aloe vera
- 1-inch ginger slice
- 1 cup grapefruit (peeled and flashes)
- 2 tablespoons honey
- 1 cup crushed ice

Methods:

A. In a blender, add all the ingredients and blend until smooth. 15

B. Strain the extract and discard the residue.

C. Pour into serving glasses and serve immediately.

6. Dill and Carrot Salad

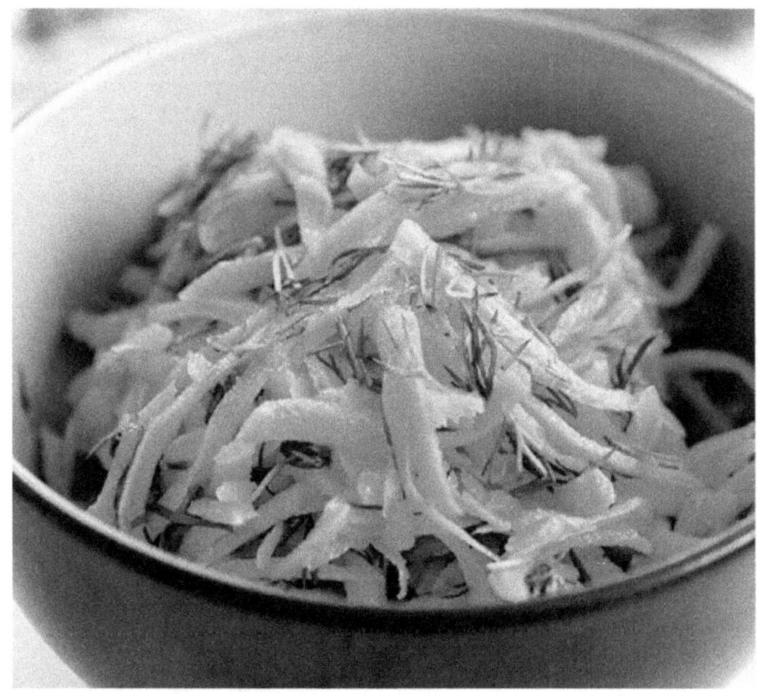

Preparation time: 5 minutes

Yield: 2 servings

The list of ingredients:

- 1 tablespoon chopped dill
- 3 carrots (peeled and grated)
- 1 tablespoons vinegar
- 2 tablespoons lemon juice

Methods:

A. On a platter, add the carrots, lemon juice, and vinegar then toss to combine.

B. Sprinkle dill on top and serve.

C. Enjoy.

7. Bone Broth

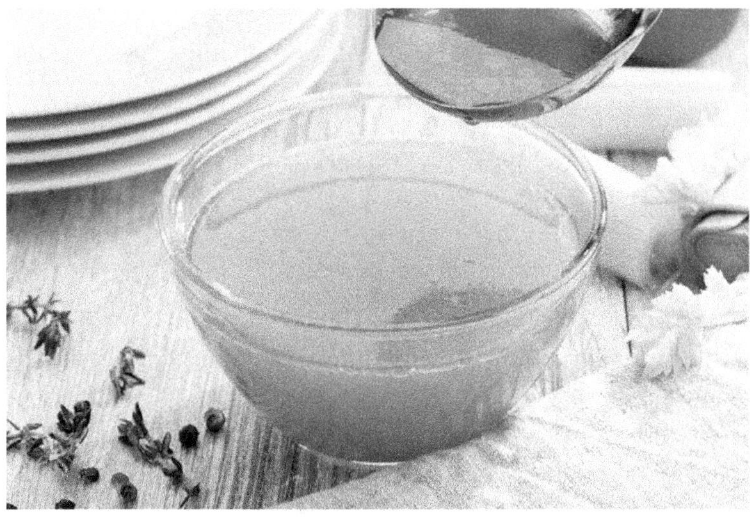

Preparation time: 2 hours

Yield: 5 servings

The list of ingredients:

- 1 tablespoon cooking oil
- 5 cups water
- 1/2 teaspoon salt
- 1 onion (sliced)
- 1 oz. bone (cleaned)
- 1-inch ginger slice
- 5-6 garlic cloves

- 1/2 teaspoon white pepper

- 2 tablespoons apple cider vinegar

Methods:

A. In a large skillet, add the bones, water, onion, garlic, ginger, oil, vinegar, salt, and pepper then stir. Cover with the lid.
B. Leave to cook on a low heat for 2 hours.
C. Strain the broth and discard the residue.
D. Serve hot and enjoy.

8. Grilled Salmon

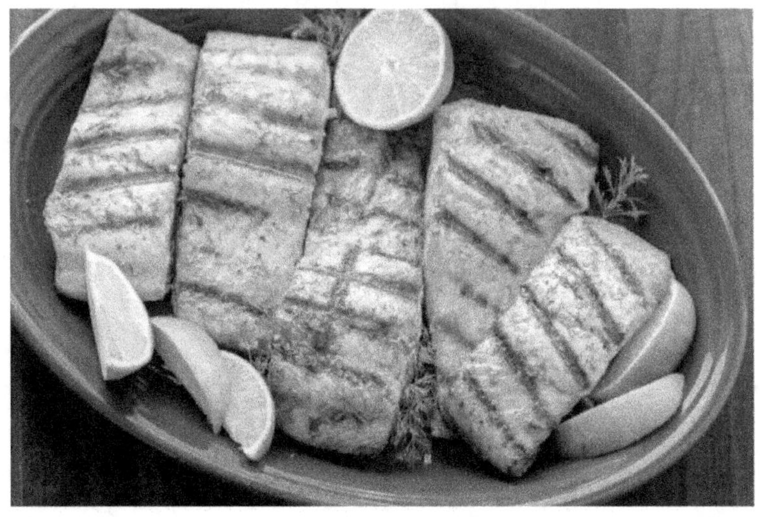

Preparation time: 35 minutes

Yield: 2 servings

The list of ingredients:

- 2 tablespoons olive oil
- 1 teaspoon fish sauce
- 2 salmon fillets
- 1/2 teaspoon black pepper
- 1/2 teaspoon garlic paste
- 1/2 teaspoon oregano
- 1 teaspoon salt

- 1/4 teaspoon turmeric powder

- 3 tablespoons lemon juice

Methods:

A. Sprinkle turmeric powder on fish and rub it in all over.

B. Leave it for 10-15 minutes before washing the fish well.

C. In a bowl, add the vinegar, lemon juice, pepper, salt, fish sauce, and oregano then toss to combine.

D. Spread the mixture on the fish fillets and rub it in with your hands.

E. Preheat the grill and spray it with oil.

F. Place the fish fillets on the grill and cook until they brown well.

G. Flip them over and make sure both sides are cooked well.

H. Serve and enjoy.

9. Shrimp Salad with Mint Dressing

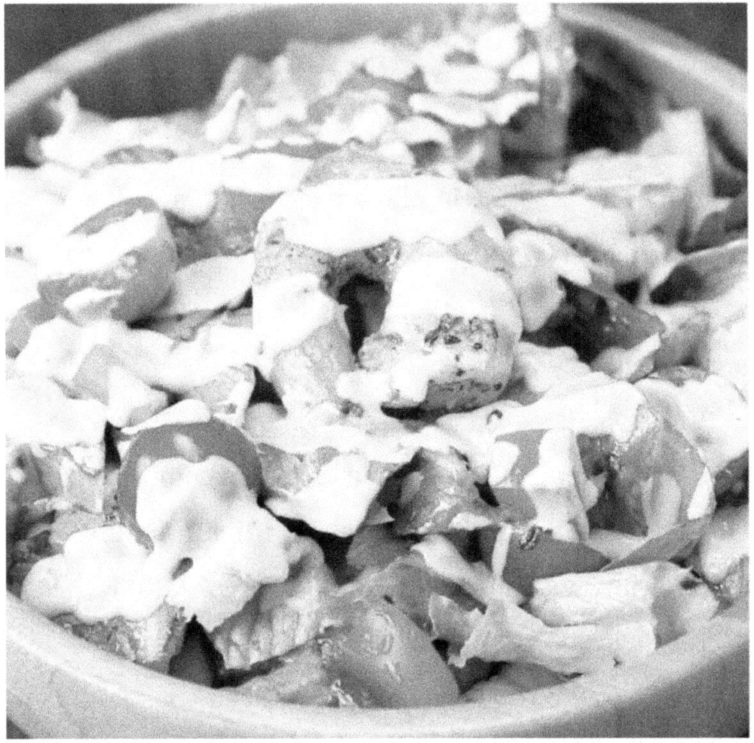

Preparation time: 25 minutes

Yield: 3 servings

The list of ingredients:

- 2 tablespoons olive oil
- 2 carrots (shredded)
- 2 tablespoons lemon juice

- 1 bunch mint leaves

- 1/4 teaspoon salt

- 1 cup coconut milk

- 1 green chili

- 2-3 garlic cloves (minced)

- 2 avocados, pitted (chopped)

- 1/2 teaspoon black pepper

- 1 oz. shrimps

- 1 bunch kale leaves (chopped)

Methods:

A. In a blender, add the coconut milk, green chili, lemon juice, and mint leaves then blend well.

B. Heat the oil in a saucepan and sauté the shrimp for 5 minutes.

C. Season with salt and pepper.

D. Remove from the heat and transfer into a serving dish with carrots, avocado, and kale.

E. Serve the salad with mint dressing and enjoy.

10. Tomato & Cucumber Salad

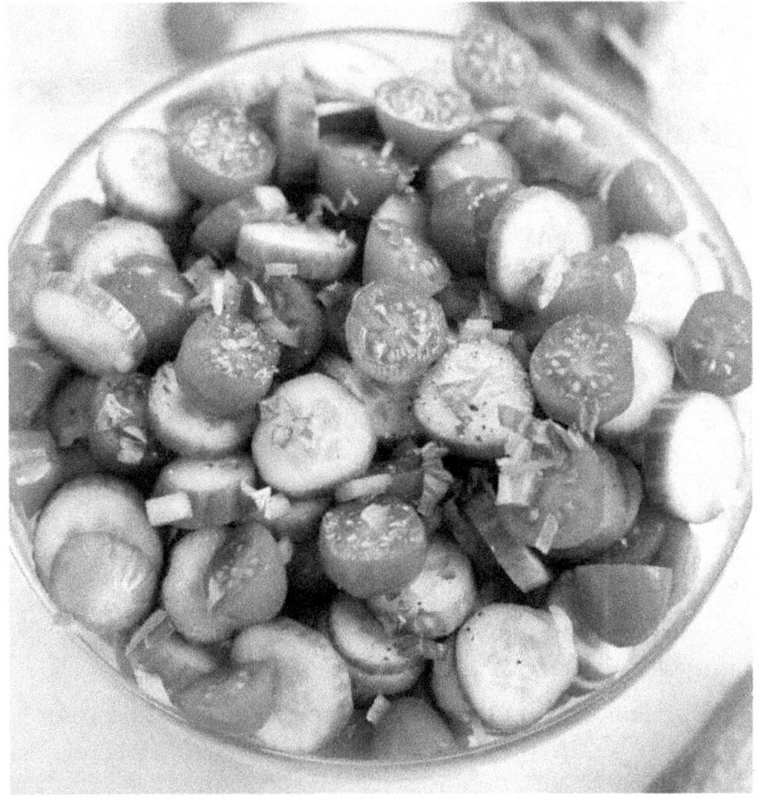

Preparation time: 5 minutes

Yield: 2 servings

The list of ingredients:

- 2 tablespoons lemon juice
- 1/4 teaspoon cinnamon powder

- 2 tomatoes (chopped)
- 1/4 teaspoon black pepper
- 2 tablespoons apple cider vinegar
- 1 cucumber (peeled and chopped)
- 1/4 teaspoon salt
- 1 onion (sliced)

Methods:

A. In a bowl, add all the ingredients and toss to combine.
B. Transfer to a serving dish.
C. Serve and enjoy.

11. Cherry Pomegranate Punch

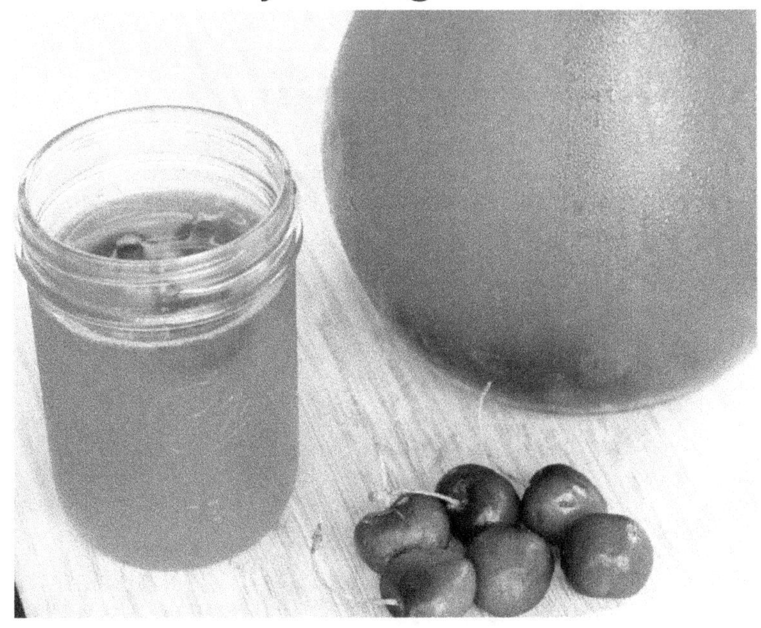

Preparation time: 10 minutes

Yield: 2 servings

The list of ingredients:

- 2 mint leaves
- 2 cups pomegranate seeds
- 1/2 cup cherry juice (no sugar added)
- 1-inch ginger slice
- 1 cup ice chunks

Methods:

A. In a blender, add all the ingredients and blend well.

B. Strain the juice and discard the residue.

C. Add to serving glasses and serve.

12. Stir-Fried Zucchini with Ground Beef

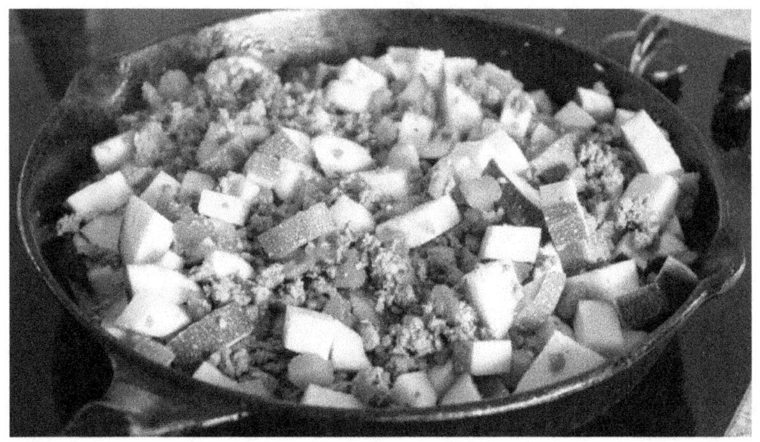

Preparation time: 25 minutes

Yield: 3 servings

The list of ingredients:

- 1/2 teaspoons ground cumin seeds
- 1/4 teaspoon salt
- 1 onion (sliced)
- 1/2 cup chicken broth
- 1/4 teaspoons cumin powder
- 2 tablespoons coconut oil
- 2 zucchinis (sliced)

- 2 tablespoons vinegar

- 1/2 teaspoon garlic paste

- 1 ounce beef mince

- 1/4 teaspoon chili powder

Methods:

A. Heat the oil in a pan and sauté the garlic and onion for 1 minute.

B. Add the beef mince and fry until nicely browned.

C. Add the zucchini and stir well.

D. Fry for 5 minutes on medium heat.

E. Add in the chicken broth, salt, chili powder, and vinegar then cook on low heat for 10-15 minutes.

F. When all the water is absorbed add the cumin and cinnamon powder then stir well.

G. Serve and enjoy.

13. Egg & Garden Salad

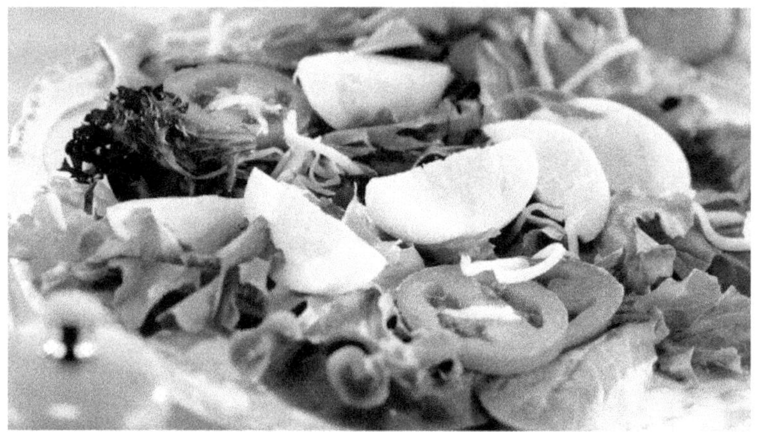

Preparation time: 15 minutes

Yield: 3 servings

The list of ingredients:

- 3 lettuce leaves (sliced)
- 1 cup cabbages (chopped)
- 1 teaspoon salt
- 1 cup broccoli florets
- 2 tomatoes (chopped)
- 1 carrot (sliced)
- 3 boiled eggs (sliced)
- 1/2 teaspoon black pepper

Methods:

A. In a large bowl, add the tomatoes, broccoli, carrots, lettuce, and cabbage then toss to combine.

B. Place the egg slices on top and season with salt and pepper.

C. Enjoy.

14. Ginger-Zest and Watermelon Shrub

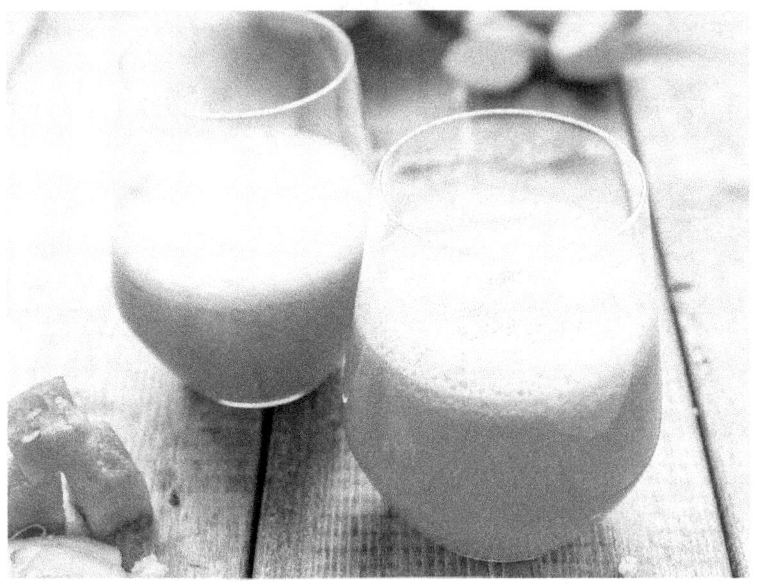

Preparation time: 10 minutes

Yield: 2 servings

The list of ingredients:

- 1-inch ginger slice
- 2 cups watermelon chunks (seeded)
- 1 cup ice chunks
- 2 tablespoons lemon juice
- 1 cup water

Methods:

A. In a juicer, add all the ingredients and blend well.

B. Add to serving glasses and serve.

15. Poached Eggs in Tomato Sauce

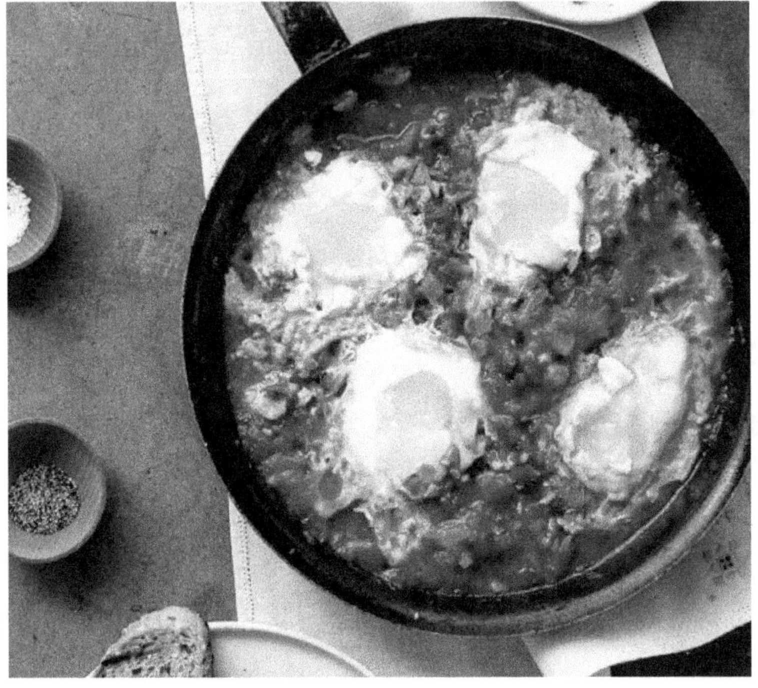

Preparation time: 35 minutes

Yield: 4 servings

The list of ingredients:

- 1 cup tomato sauce
- 2 tablespoons olive oil
- 1 teaspoon salt
- 1 cup tomato puree

- 1 onion (sliced)
- 1/2 teaspoon black pepper
- 1 onion (chopped)
- 4 eggs

Methods:

A. Heat the oil in a pan and sauté the onion for 1-2 minutes.
B. Add the tomato puree and tomato sauce then fry for 10-15 minutes.
C. Create four, small wells in the tomato gravy and crack an egg into each well.
D. Cover with a lid and cook on low heat for 10 minutes.
E. Sprinkle salt and pepper on top.
F. Serve and enjoy.

16. Coco - Banana Milkshake

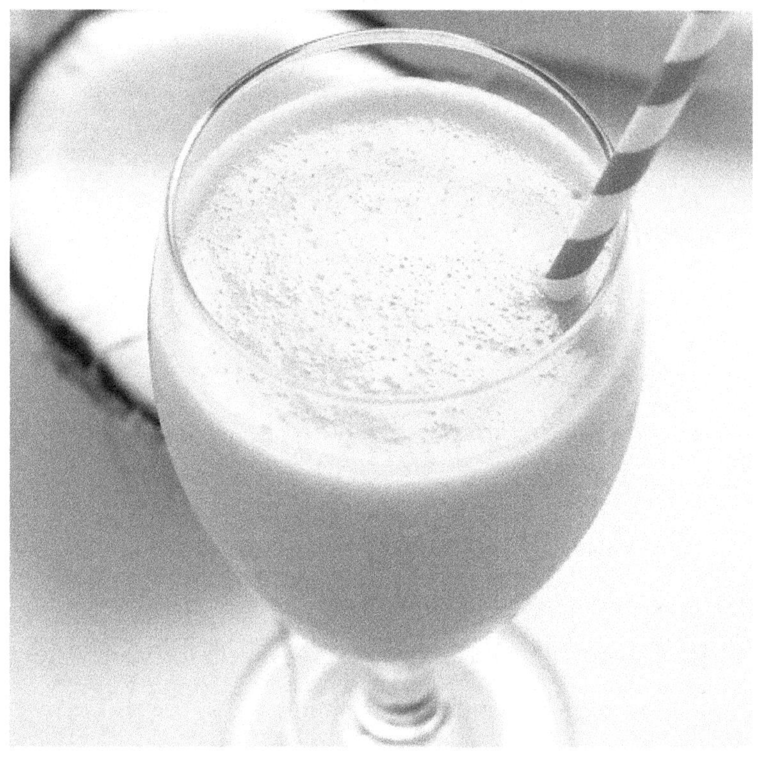

Preparation time: 5 minutes

Yield: 1 servings

The list of ingredients:

- 2 tablespoons brown sugar
- 1 cup coconut milk
- 7 ice cubes

- 2 ripe bananas

- 1/4 teaspoon cardamom powder

Methods:

A. In a blender, add the coconut milk, cardamom powder, brown sugar, and bananas then blend well.

B. Pour into a glass and add the ice chunks.

C. Serve and enjoy.

17. Citrusy Radish Salad

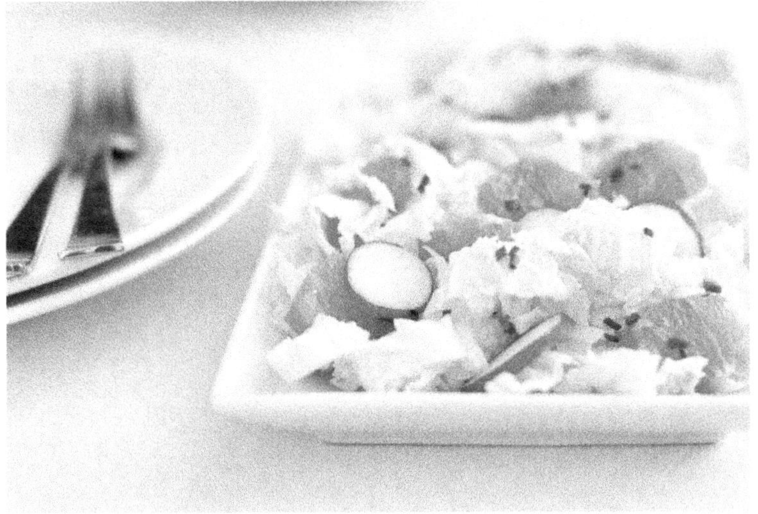

Preparation time: 10 minutes

Yield: 3 servings

The list of ingredients:

- 1 cup grapefruit flashes (peeled)
- 1 teaspoon fresh dill (chopped)
- 1 cup cabbage (chopped)
- 2 tablespoons apple cider vinegar
- 1/2 cup pineapple juice
- 1 radish (sliced)
- 1 pinch of salt

Methods:

A. In a medium bowl, add the pineapple juice, vinegar, and salt.

B. Add the cabbage, radish, and grapefruit then toss to combine.

C. Sprinkle dill on top.

D. Serve and enjoy.

18. Cucumber, Avocado, and Dill Smoothie

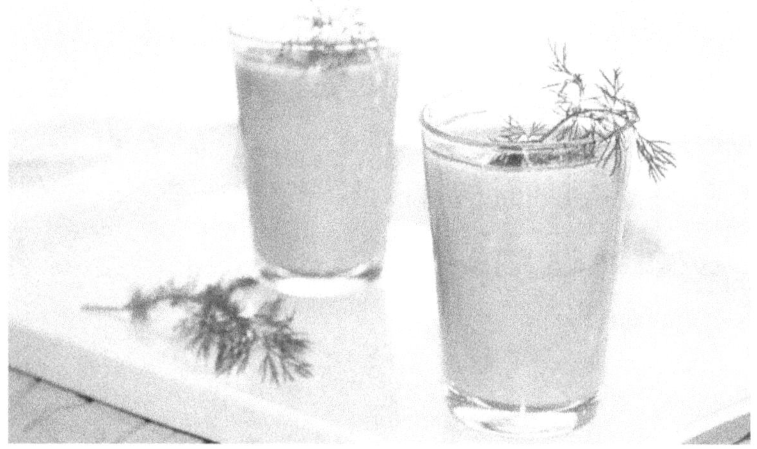

Preparation time: 5 minutes

Yield: 2 servings

The list of ingredients:

- 1 cup coconut milk
- 2 tablespoons dill (chopped)
- 2 kiwis (peeled and sliced)
- 1 avocado (pitted)
- 1 teaspoon coconut (shredded)
- 1 cucumber (peeled and sliced)
- 2 tablespoons lemon juice

Methods:

A. In a blender add all the ingredients and blend well.

B. Drain the extract and discard the residue.

C. Serve and enjoy.

19. Stewed Beef and Mushrooms

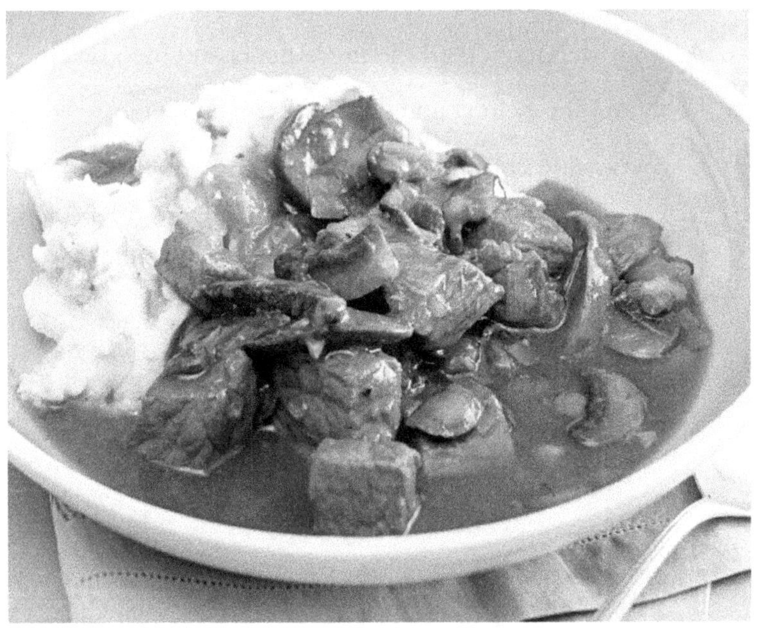

Preparation time: 1 hour 15 minutes

Yield: 3 servings

The list of ingredients:

- 1 bay leaf
- 1 cup mushrooms (sliced)
- 1/2 teaspoon black pepper
- 1/4 teaspoon cumin powder
- 4-5 garlic cloves (minced)

- 1 clove
- 3 tablespoons oil
- 1 onion (sliced)
- 1 ounce beef meat
- 4 cups water

Methods:

A. Heat the oil in a skillet, add the mushrooms, and fry for 5 minutes. Set aside.

B. In the same skillet, add the onion, bay leaf, and clove then sauté for 1-2 minutes.

C. Add the beef and garlic, and fry until browned.

D. Add the water and cook on low heat for 1 hour.

E. Transfer the fried mushrooms, salt, pepper, and cumin powder and stir well.

F. Discard the bay leaf and cook for 10 more minutes.

G. Serve hot and enjoy.

20. Roasted Chicken

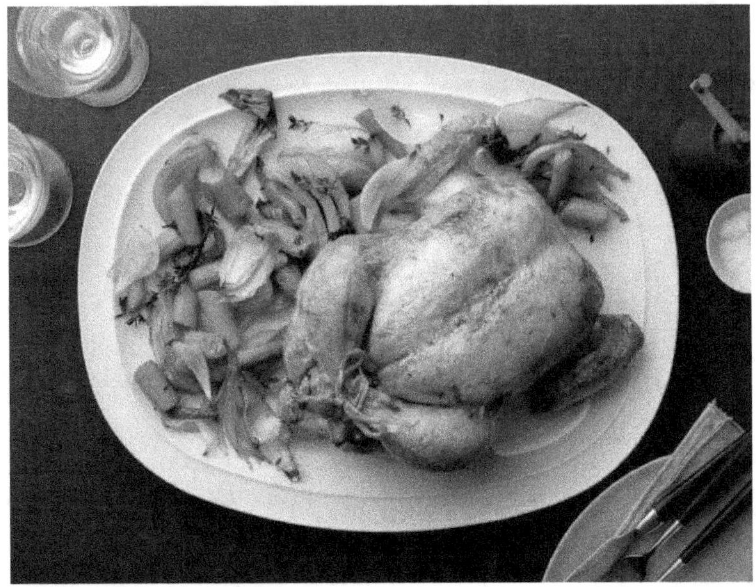

Preparation time: 40 minutes

Yield: 6 servings

The list of ingredients:

- 2 tablespoons lemon juice
- 1/2 teaspoon garlic paste
- 1/2 teaspoon black pepper
- 3 tablespoons vinegar
- 1/2 teaspoon salt

- 1 whole chicken

- 1 tablespoon dried rosemary

- 2 tablespoons olive oil

- 1/4 teaspoon sea salt

- 1/2 cup orange juice (no sugar added)

- 1/2 teaspoon cinnamon powder

- 2 tablespoons fish sauce

- 1/2 teaspoon ginger paste

Methods:

A. Preheat the oven to 355 degrees F.

B. In a bowl, add the orange juice, rosemary, oil, lemon juice, vinegar, ginger paste, garlic paste, fish sauce, salt, pepper, and rosemary then mix well.

C. Rub this mixture into the chicken thoroughly.

D. Place the chicken in a greased pan and bake for 30-35 minutes or until golden brown.

21. Strawberry and Cherry Shake

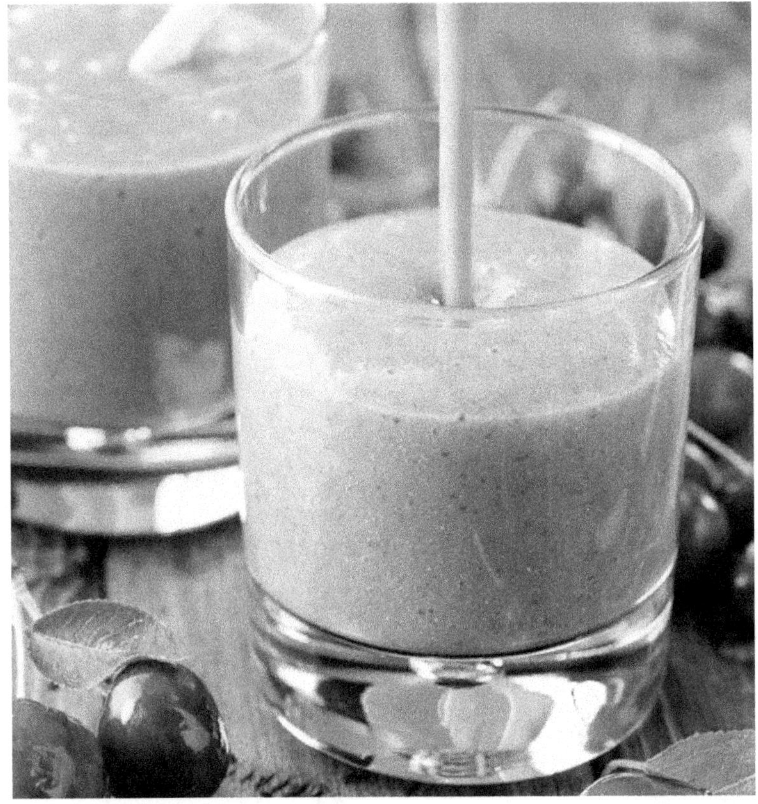

Preparation time: 5 minutes

Yield: 2 servings

The list of ingredients:

- 1 cup almond milk
- 1 cup strawberries

- Few ice chunks (about 6)
- 1 cup cherries
- 1/2 cup coconut milk

Methods:

A. In a blender add all the ingredients and blend well.
B. Serve and enjoy.

22. Seasonal Breakfast Fruit Bowl

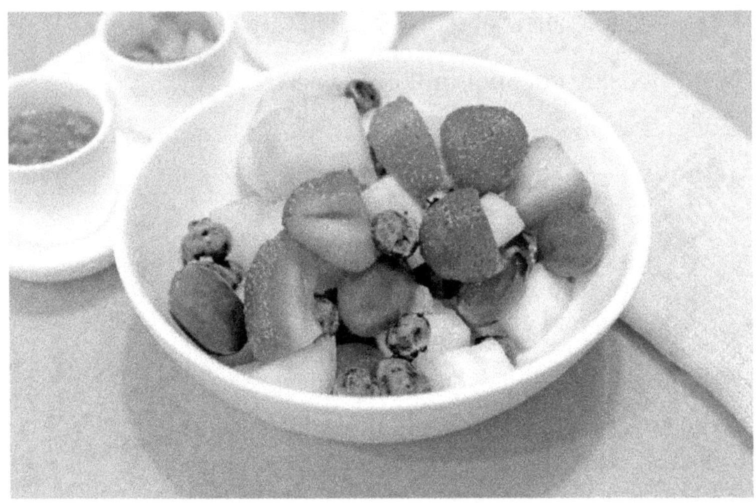

Preparation time: 5 minutes

Yield: 3 servings

The list of ingredients:

- 1 orange (peeled)
- 2-3 mint leaves chopped
- 2 kiwis (sliced)
- 2 bananas (sliced)
- 1/4 teaspoon Dijon mustard powder
- 2 tablespoons lime juice
- 1 cup pineapple chunks

- 1/2 cup pineapple juice

- 1/2 cup strawberries (sliced)

Methods:

A. In a bowl, add all the fruits and toss to combine.

B. In another bowl, add the lime juice, pineapple juice, mint leaves, and mustard powder then mix.

C. Pour this mixture over the fruits and toss.

D. Enjoy.

23. Chicken Mince with Peas

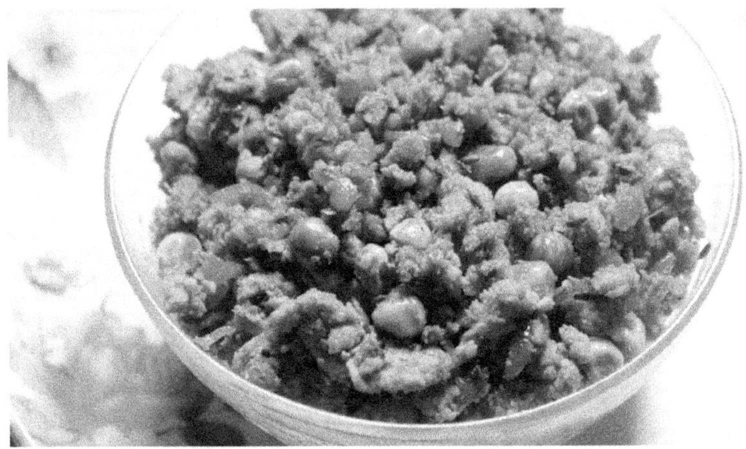

Preparation time: 35 minutes

Yield: 4 servings

The list of ingredients:

- 1 bunch fresh coriander (chopped)
- 1/2 teaspoon chili powder
- 1 oz. minced chicken
- 1/4 teaspoon turmeric powder
- 1/2 teaspoon cumin powder
- 1/4 teaspoon garlic paste
- 2 green chilies
- 1 onion (chopped)

- 2 cups chicken broth

- 2 tablespoons olive oil

- 1/2 teaspoon cinnamon powder

- 1/4 teaspoon salt

- 1 cup peas

- 1 lemon

- 1 cup tomato puree

Methods:

A. Heat the oil in a pan, add the onion then fry for 2 minutes.

B. Add the chicken mince and garlic and fry until golden.

C. Add the tomato puree and fry again for 5-10 minutes.

D. Add salt, chili powder, turmeric powder, and peas then fry for 5 minutes.

E. Add the chicken broth and cover the pan with a lid. Cook on a low heat for 15 minutes.

F. Sprinkle in the cumin and cinnamon powder.

G. Transfer to serving dish and top with the coriander and green chilies.

H. Squeeze some lemon juice over the top.

I. Serve and enjoy.

24. Curried Eggs

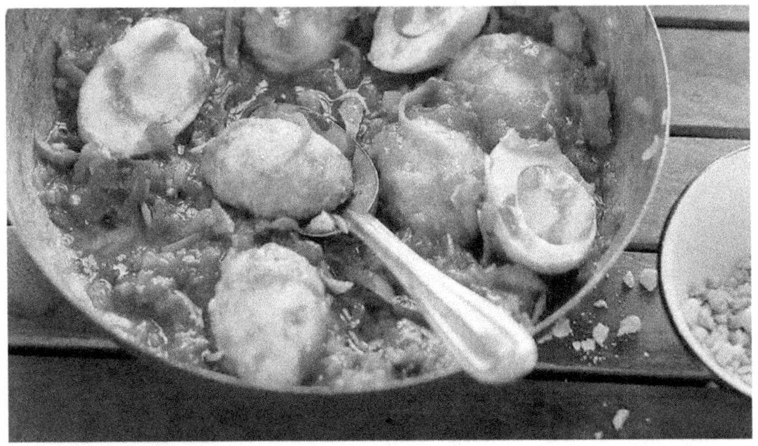

Preparation time: 35 minutes

Yield: 3 servings

The list of ingredients:

- 1 onion (chopped)
- 2 eggs (hard boiled (halved))
- 2 tablespoons olive oil
- 1 teaspoon salt
- 1/2 teaspoon cumin powder
- 1 onion (sliced)
- 1/4 cup water
- 1/2 teaspoon black pepper

- 1/4 teaspoon cinnamon powder

- 1 cup tomato puree

Methods:

A. Heat the oil in a pan and sauté the onion for 1-2 minutes.

B. Add the tomato puree and fry for 10-15 minutes.

C. Add the water, bring to a boil, reduce, and cook for 5-10 minutes.

D. When the water has been absorbed, add the salt, pepper, cumin powder, and cinnamon powder and mix well.

E. Add the eggs and toss to combine.

F. Serve hot and enjoy.

25. Green Salsa

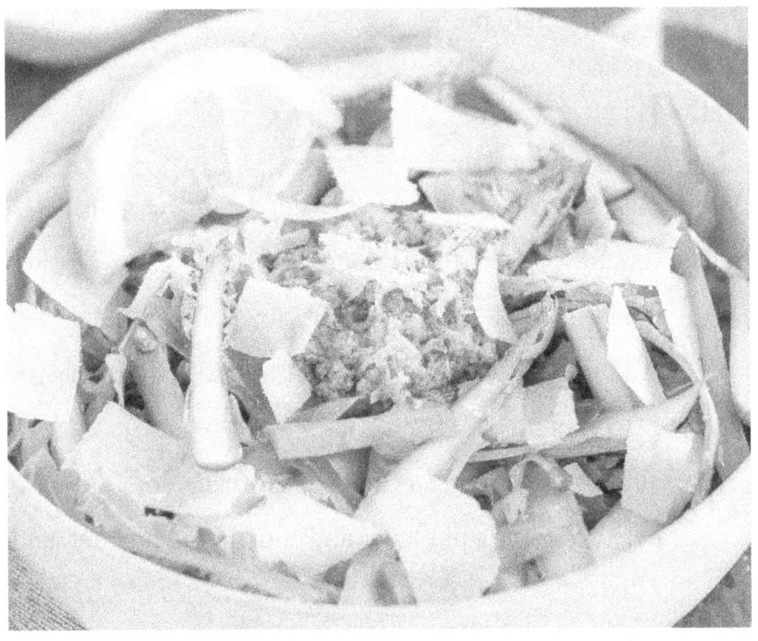

Preparation time: 15 minutes

Yield: 3 servings

The list of ingredients:

- 1/4 teaspoon Dijon mustard powder
- 1 oz. asparagus (cut into ribbons)
- 1 tablespoons freshly chopped dill
- 2 fennel bulbs (sliced)
- 2 tablespoons lime juice

Methods:

A. In a medium bowl, add all the ingredients and toss to combine.

B. Serve and enjoy.

26. Banana Pancakes

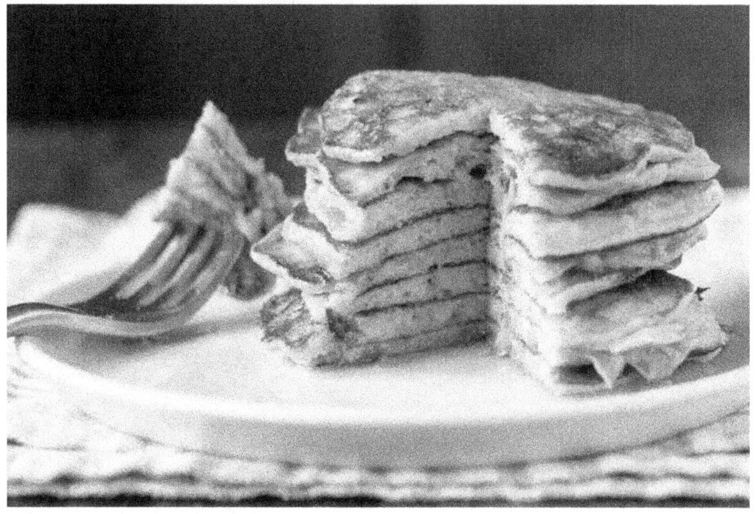

Preparation time: 30 minutes

Yield: 1 serving

The list of ingredients:

- 2 large, whisked eggs
- 1 tablespoon butter (for the pan)
- 1 medium, mashed ripe banana

Methods:

A. In a medium bowl, mix the mashed bananas and whisked eggs together.

A. In a medium bowl, mix the mashed bananas and whisked eggs together.

B. Heat your griddle pan over the medium heat and grease it with the butter.

C. Drop 2 tablespoon portions of the batter onto the hot griddle and allow it to cook for about a minute or until it bubbles on top slightly.

D. Flip and cook until it browns on the other side.

E. Serve and enjoy!

27. Vegetable Stew

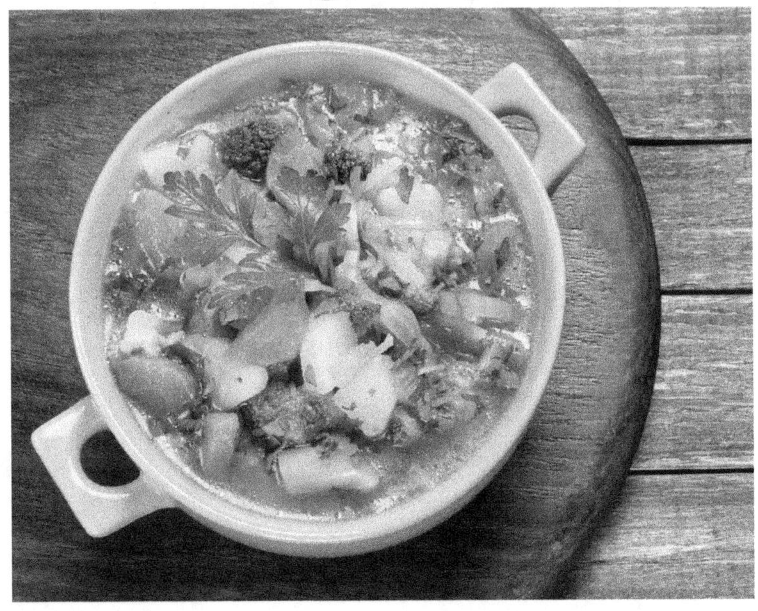

Preparation time: 45 minutes

Yield: 4 servings

The list of ingredients:

- 1/2 teaspoon black pepper
- 2-3 garlic cloves (minced)
- 3 cup chicken broth
- 1 teaspoon salt
- 1 cup water

- 2 carrots (peppered and sliced)
- 1 onion (sliced)
- 1 cup broccoli florets
- 2 tablespoons olive oil

Methods:

A. Heat the oil in a skillet and sauté the onion for about 2 minutes.

B. Add the garlic and then stir for 30 seconds.

C. Add the carrots and broccoli and sauté for 5-10 minutes on medium heat.

D. Add the water, chicken broth, salt, and pepper then stir.

E. Cover with a lid and leave to cook on low heat for 25-30 minutes.

F. Serve and enjoy.

28. Colourful Fruit Bowl

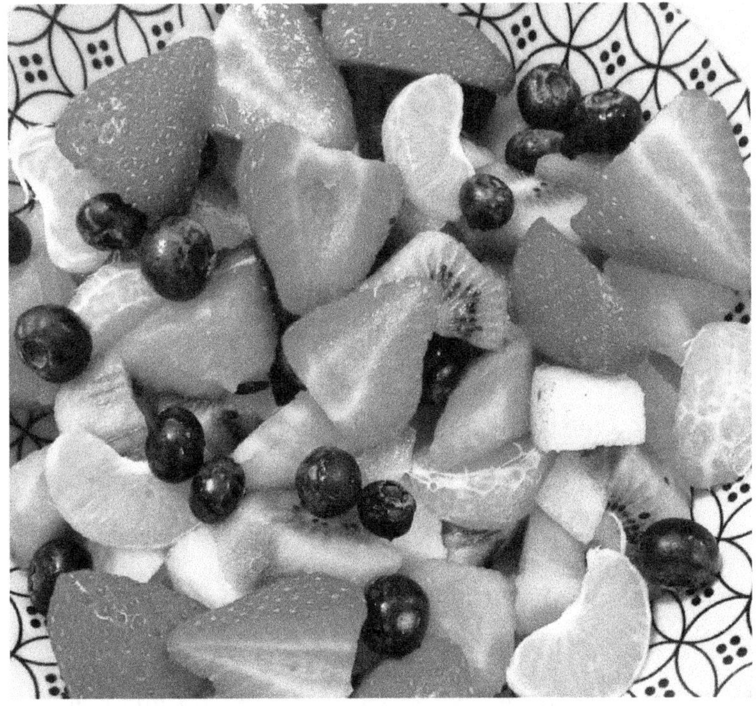

Preparation time: 10 minutes

Yield: 3 servings

The list of ingredients:

- 1 cup strawberries (halved)
- 2 oranges (peeled)
- 2 bananas (sliced)

- 1 cup grapes

- 2 tablespoons lemon juice

- 1 cup pineapple (chunks)

Methods:

A. In a bowl, add all the fruits and toss to combine.

B. Drizzle lemon juice on top and serve.

29. Chicken-Stuffed Bell Peppers

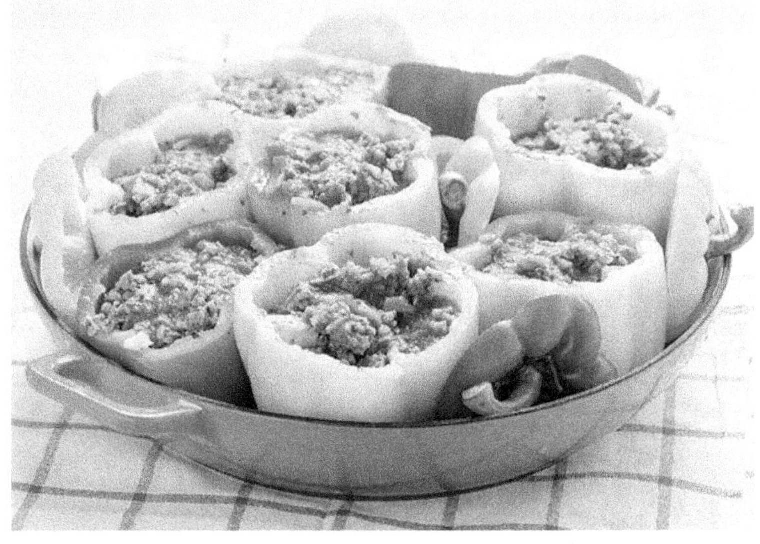

Preparation time: 35 minutes

Yield: 4 servings

The list of ingredients:

- 1/4 teaspoon garlic paste
- 2 yellow bell peppers (make a cut from the stem)
- 2 tablespoons olive oil
- 1/2 cup tomato puree
- 1/4 teaspoon salt
- 1 cup chicken mince

- 2 red bell peppers (make a cut from the stem)
- 1/2 teaspoon black pepper

Methods:

A. Heat oil in a pan, add the garlic then fry for 1 minute.

B. Add the chicken mince and stir well.

C. When the chicken mince becomes golden brown, add the tomato puree and fry again for 5-10 minutes.

D. Season with salt and pepper.

E. Preheat the oven to 355 degrees F.

F. Fill the bell peppers with fried mince and place into the greased pan.

G. Bake for 10 minutes.

H. Serve and enjoy.

30. Spinach & Kale Smoothie

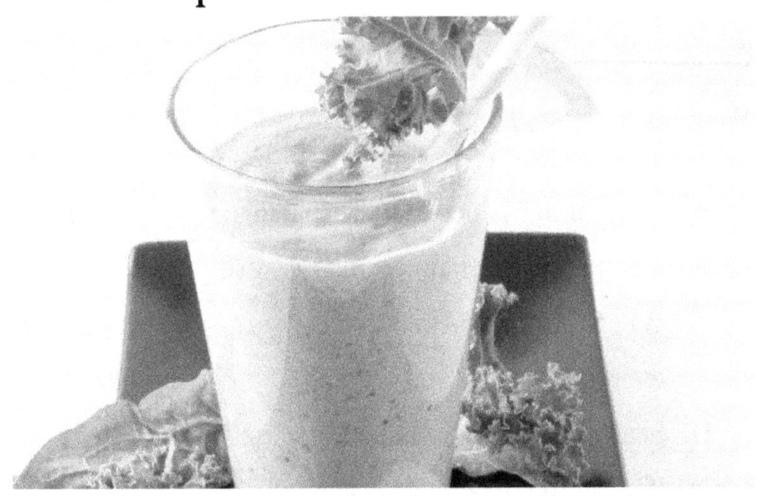

Preparation time: 5 minutes

Yield: 3 servings

The list of ingredients:

- 2 tablespoons lime juice
- 1 cup grapes
- 1 cup ice
- 1 cup kale (chopped)
- 1 cup pineapple juice
- 2 mint leaves
- 1 cup baby spinach leaves

Methods:

A. In a blender add all the ingredients and blend until smooth.

B. Transfer to serving glasses.

C. Serve and enjoy.